31 Ways to Self-Care

ANDREA JOYCE

Copyright © 2021 Andrea Joyce

All rights reserved.

All rights reserved. No part of this book may be reproduced in any form or by any means without the prior written consent of the Publisher, excepting brief quotes used in reviews.

ISBN: 9798745250484

DEDICATION

For my niece, Keyauna Cameron Bowman, the amazing young woman who taught me what self-care is and why it is so important. Your growth and maturity are very inspiring. I love you.

For my three heartbeats, Icis, DeAngelo and Danielle, you are all overcomers. You survived and flourished even without fathers in your lives. I cannot wait to see how much you accomplish and how far God will take you. I am very proud of you.
I love you.

And for my mother, Marjorie Cameron, you have always been a strong example of not giving up. You have always encouraged me to do the right thing even when it did not feel right. You always told me when I was right and when I was wrong, You never let me skate by just doing the bare minimum. You pushed me to be better than I thought I was, You taught me to have faith in God and you taught me how to forgive. I am the woman I am because of you.
I love you.

FOREWORD

This has not been a peaceful time in our lives. With a pandemic and natural disasters happening across the world, it has been hard to get back to business as usual. We are wearing physical masks like decorations. We cannot be close to anyone anymore, and the little things we took for granted we can no longer do. It has taken a toll on our personal life, our professional life, and our mental and physical health.

Even though we have these heartbreaking events going on around us, we must remember that life is worth living and we matter. I wanted to write this book to share with you some things to do to heal from the state of the world. You, above all, must be healthy so you can continue to live. Self-care is so important. Getting your mental, physical, emotional, spiritual, financial, and relational health in order is a priority even as the world throws curve ball after curve ball.

I have shared some things I do to get myself on track. My sister gave me a suggestion. She suggested that every morning after I wake up, I look in the mirror and decide one thing that I will do for my self-care. I have taken that to heart. I challenge you to do the same. The way you start your morning is how your day will continue. It is up to you to prioritize yourself and shape your day the way you want it to go.

This journal is your personal and private safe place. Be open and honest. You are on course to becoming healthier. It has been set up with words of encouragement, suggestions, questions for you to think about and answer, and a scripture to meditate on. I hope it will change you for the better and that these activities will become habits you use throughout your life.

Andrea Joyce

ACKNOWLEDGMENTS

April 2021

Foremost, I want to thank my Father, God, for blessing me to write this book. I am grateful to have the opportunity to share my thoughts and feelings.

With much appreciation to:

My mother, Marjorie Cameron, for encouraging me and always being someone I could depend on. I love you, Mommy.

My children, Icis, DeAngelo, and Danielle, for inspiring me to not give up and for being patient while I wrote for hours. Thank you for your unfailing love.

My sister Regina Cameron, an awesome author who would not let me quit. Thank you for always encouraging me, sis. Your books are going to take the world by storm. I love you Wonder Twin.

My best friend/cousin/sister, Eutopia Nicole, an amazing author who kept pushing me even when I begged her to leave me alone. Thank you for your bullying tactics and your tenacity. I cannot wait for your books to come out so I can celebrate you! I love you, couster.

My best friend, Shenneace Lytle, for always motivating and supporting me. This is just the beginning, there is more in store! I love you.

My brother, Duane Cameron, you have always been a wholehearted supporter and inspiration. Thanks for always lifting me up! I love you.

My family, thank you to my aunts and uncles, Ruby, Rosa Belle, Mae Frances, Ricky, and Ted. I owe an enormous debt of gratitude to my family that has gone from here, my Daddy Daniel, my Father James, my grandparents, John, Clara, Daniel, Chrystallia, Peter, and Mary, my aunts and uncles, Phyllis, Albert, Mary, Ed, Georgianna, Frances, Edwin, Jacqueline, Thomas, Cobra, my family-friends Eva, Charlotte, Reginald, Rev. Richardson, rest in glory. You are truly missed. I have been blessed to have been raised by three sides of family. Thank you to all my nieces, nephews, and cousins, the Stradford family, the Carr family, and the Cameron/Christopher family for all your love throughout my life. You are all awesome and amazing. I love you.

My friends, you have been true blue throughout the years. Thank you to all my adopted/surrogate/spiritual mothers, fathers, aunts, uncles, sisters, brothers, children, nieces, nephews, and cousins. I want to especially give love to the Brown family. Thank you for taking me and my children into your homes and hearts. Thank you for everything. I love you.

My mentors, professional and spiritual, that have guided and advised me throughout my life. Thank you for your belief in me. Thank you for your prayers, and thank you for pouring into me. I want to send a special thank you to "Ma" Rosetta Collins. Thank you for placing your mantle upon me and pouring your wisdom into me. I will be forever grateful.

Pastor Michael D. McDuffie, Lady Jamie McDuffie, and the Mighty Sons of God Fellowship Church, words cannot express the love and gratitude I have for you. You taught me, nurtured me, groomed me, and pushed me to be better. I love you.

Pastor Q. Gadson, and the Believers House for giving my children and me the Word, love, help, and correction. I appreciate learning from each and every one of you. Thank you to my spiritual mother, Elder Marilyn Morrison, "Pop" Morrison and Angela Stewart, for how you have blessed the children and me, time and time again. I am honored to be a member of such an uplifting and wonderful church.

I want to acknowledge two special, talented women who are not only family, who are not only friends, but have always been my confidants, who have wiped many tears from my eyes, who have been there throughout every loss I have faced. You have taught me the meaning of true, unconditional love and showed what being a strong, confidant woman is. I love you to the moon and beyond. Thank you Habibah Abdul Shaheed and Izora "Bonnie" Carr Duck. This success is our success!

I am grateful and appreciative to Lady Ty the Great, Ty Johnson, for being such an awesome coach. Thank you for taking the time to share your wisdom with the Triumph Over Trauma (T.O.T.S.) group. Thank you for making a way for me to get into your class, so I could begin and complete this journey. I look forward to the next level. I thank God for you. Thank you to the T.O.T.S. team, Vadine Chandler and Jannine Swersky for making sure we were always on point. Thank you and Congratulations to my fellow T.O.T.S. authors, we made it! Thank you to the GREATS for all your wisdom, guidance, and support.

Last but not least, to my heroes, you the readers. Without you I could not do this. I am grateful for your support! I pray this book will help bring about breakthrough, healing, and blessing in your lives. I love and appreciate you!

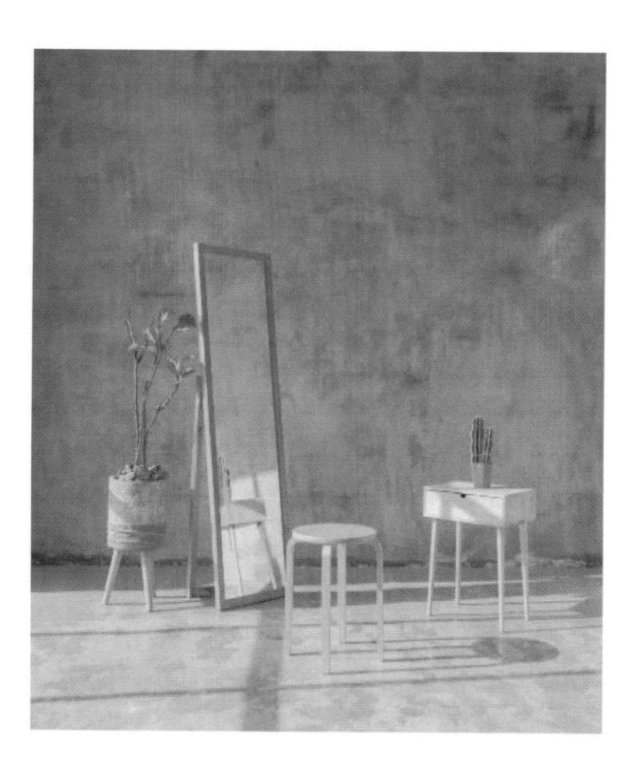

SEE YOURSELF

Are you the same person you were five years ago, five months ago, or even five minutes ago? Rushing to get to work, getting children ready for school and constantly moving does not allow for time to see who we are. Even though there are mirrors around, how often do we take the time to evaluate our eyes, our noses, our teeth, our faces, or our bodies? Science says that every seven years we change physically, we mature. The you that you were at 14, is not the you that you were at 21 or 28. Filters and photo shopping even make our pictures an unreliable source of what we look like.

You need to become familiar with who you are now. It is time to take an intimate look at you. Spend at least 15 minutes looking into a mirror. Notice your face, are there any new lines or shadings? Do you have freckles or moles? Also take this time to look at your full body. Become intimate with how your body looks.

1. What do you see?_____
   _____
   _____

2. What has changed?_____
   _____
   _____

3. What do you like?_____
   _____
   _____

4. What would you like to change? _____
_____
_____

∞ ∞ ∞

Scripture verse:
"Examine yourselves, to see whether you are in the faith. Test yourselves."
2 Corinthians 13:5

This is your mirror. Draw what you see about yourself that you like.

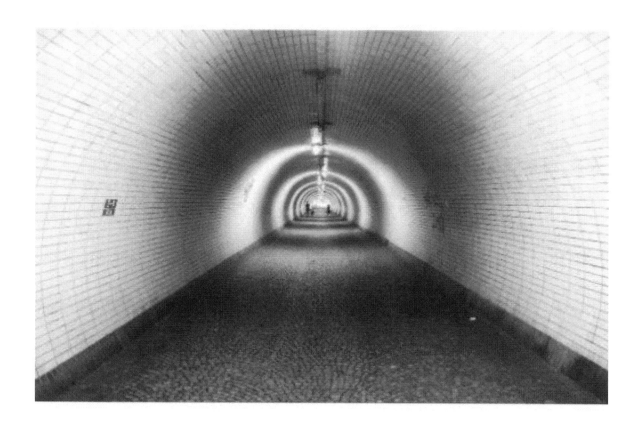

LOOK INSIDE

We sometimes get so caught up by outer appearance that we neglect our inner self. Do you notice that there are times you cry for no reason? Have you suffered from anger, anxiety, or depression? Are you mourning or grieving? Are you feeling accomplished and productive? It is so important that we care for our inner selves as much or more than our outer selves.

When was the last time you took stock of your feelings? Do not let anyone tell you how you should feel about a matter. Do not let anyone tell you how long you should stay in your feelings.

1. How are you feeling? _____
   _____
   _____

2. Is there anything affecting you? _____
   _____
   _____

3. What would you like to change? _____
   _____
   _____

4. How can you make those changes? _____
   _____
   _____

∞ ∞ ∞

Scripture verse:
"So we do not lose heart. Though our outer self is wasting away, our inner self is being renewed day by day."
2 Corinthians 4:16

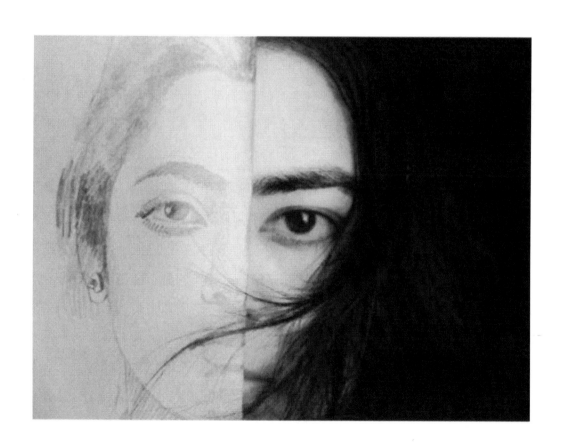

FORGIVE YOURSELF

When we look at ourselves, it may shine a light on some areas that we need to let go of. We look to ourselves to be perfect and in doing so often let ourselves down. There are areas of our lives where we feel guilty for decisions we made or did not make. We blame ourselves for mistakes and bad choices. Over time, those feelings of guilt and shame settle and fester. We wonder why we feel defeated or fearful, when new situations and opportunities are presented to us. We feel we may not deserve happiness or to be blessed with good things.

We need to let go of those feelings of unforgiveness for things we have done or allowed in our lives. Did they happen? Yes. However, we are worth forgiveness. There is nothing we can do that God will not forgive. When God forgives us, we are forgiven and can let go of the guilt, hurt, shame, disappointment, and blame.

Examine the areas of your life where you are holding unforgiveness. It is time to let go of those feelings. If you need to ask forgiveness from someone, please do. They may not be ready to forgive you, but you cannot hold on to those feelings. Ask forgiveness and let it go. If you need God to forgive you, please ask for His forgiveness and if you are sincere, He will forgive you.. Now ask yourself for forgiveness. No matter what you have said, thought or done, release yourself from the bondage of unforgiveness.

1. Are you holding something against yourself?____
_____
_____

2. Do you feel guilty about anything? _____
   _____
   _____

3. Are you ashamed of anything? _____
   _____
   _____

4. What do you need to release? _____
   _____
   _____

5. Write what you have not forgiven yourself for. This is your safe place, be as honest as you can.

   _____
   _____
   _____
   _____
   _____
   _____
   _____
   _____
   _____
   _____
   _____

6. How do you feel now that you have revealed that truth? _____
   _____
   _____

7. Ask God to help you forgive yourself. Continue working on forgiving yourself. _____

_____

_____

∞ ∞ ∞

Scripture verse:
"Lord, I prayed to you again and again, but I did not talk about my sins. So I only became weaker and more miserable. Every day you made life harder for me. I became like a dry land in the hot summertime. Selah But then I decided to confess my sins to the Lord.
I stopped hiding my guilt and told you about my sins. And you forgave them all! Selah "
Psalm 32:3-5

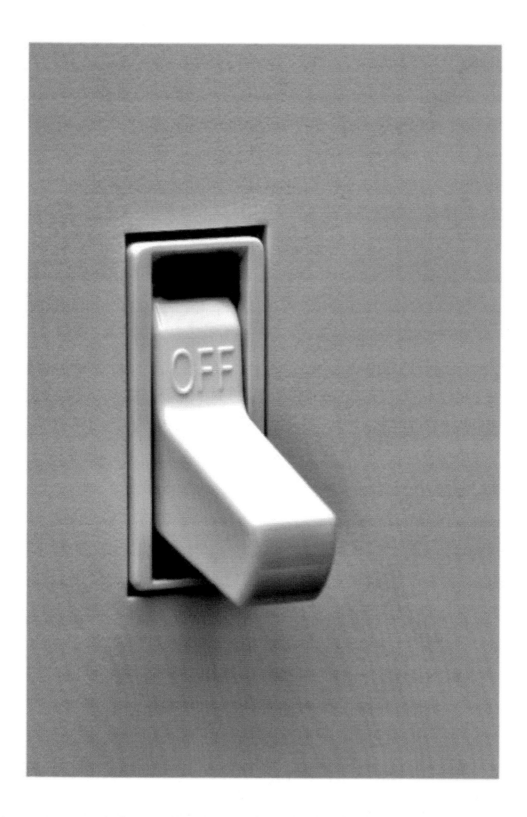

LET GO OF GRUDGES

There is a condition that feeds off us and steals our joy, takes away our hope and hinders our growth. This condition is unforgiveness. Holding onto resentment, bitterness, and grudges against someone can cause many complications in our natural and spiritual life. Grudges can cause stress and stress can cause illnesses and death.

Unforgiveness does not affect the person who has angered, hurt, betrayed, or disappointed you, it affects you. Sleepless nights, overeating, not eating, and headaches are a few symptoms of not forgiving someone. While you are up pacing, plotting, and planning against someone and wearing yourself out, they are deep in sleep or have moved on and are living their life.

Forgiving someone does not mean that they were right to do what they did or said; it means that you will not let it affect you anymore. You forgive for yourself, not others, so that you can have peace. True forgiveness means that even though you may not forget what they did, the sting of it does not hurt anymore. You will not continue rehearsing it. Though you may forgive someone, it does not mean that you must keep them in your life. It is fine to cut ties and go your separate ways.

Forgiveness may not hold the first, second or third time. Do not feel bad that you may still harbor ill feelings, continue working on forgiving. It took me over 30 years to forgive someone close to me. They never apologized, they never let me speak about my pain to them, they shut me down when I tried, but I could still forgive. I prayed and asked God to help me forgive. I prayed for God's help for a few years before I could truly forgive. I wrote a letter detailing everything that happened that hurt and angered me. I wrote it as if the person were standing in front of me. I spoke my heart and said what I needed to say the way I needed to say it. When I finished writing the letter, I read it out loud as if the person were standing there, and then I burned it. A few weeks later I knew I had forgiven them; I felt it in my heart. There are some instances where a letter will not be enough. You may have to talk to them face to face or over the phone. There are times because the person is unavailable that you can forgive on your own. Pray and ask God to reveal how you can be released from unforgiveness.

1. Are you harboring unforgiveness?_____
   _____
   _____

2. Who do you need to forgive?_____
   _____
   _____

3. What measures will you take to forgive?_____
   _____
   _____

4. Were you able to forgive and let it go?_____
   _____
   _____

∞ ∞ ∞

Scripture verse:
"*Don't be angry with each other but forgive each other. If you feel someone has wronged you, forgive them. Forgive others because the Lord forgave you.*"
Colossians 3:13

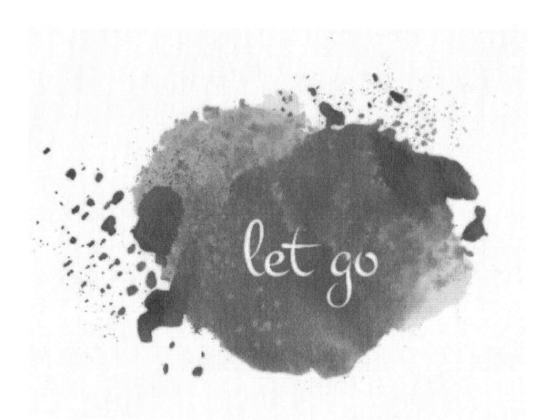

LET GO OF THE PAST

"The rear-view mirror is smaller than the front window", "the past should stay in the past" and "we don't have to be prisoners of our past" are some clichés that we hear when we talk about the past. We have been told many times that we cannot move forward if we continue holding on to the past. There are some things in our past that are holding us captive in the present, and that may cripple our futures.

We must learn to accept who we were back then and acknowledge that we are different now. There are people who have been called to do great things, but because of where they are from, how they grew up, the choices or mistakes made, they refuse to move forward. It is fruitless to continue reviewing what happened back when or wishing we could have done things differently.

There are many who feel they are not qualified to walk into their dreams because of the sins of their past. They feel they will be judged, criticized, or ridiculed, so they stay in the background afraid of what will happen if their skeletons are exposed. A mentor once told me that if you told your skeletons, the enemy could not use your past against you. You don't have to yell your mistakes and misdeeds from the rooftop, however acknowledging them when necessary, will help you get past them.

1. Is there anything you need to acknowledge?_____
   _____
   _____

2. Is there anything you need to let go?_____
   _____
   _____

3. What steps will you take to move forward? _____
_____
_____

∞ ∞ ∞

Scripture verse:
"*Brothers and sisters, I know that I still have a long way to go. But there is one thing I do: I forget what is in the past and try as hard as I can to reach the goal before me.*"
Philippians 3:13

```
┌─────────────────┐
│    REARVIEW     │
│     MIRROR      │
│     (PAST)      │
└─────────────────┘
```

```
┌─────────────────────────────────────────────┐
│                                             │
│                                             │
│              FRONT WINDOW                   │
│                                             │
│         (WHERE YOU ARE HEADED)              │
│                                             │
│                                             │
└─────────────────────────────────────────────┘
```

Both are in front of you, but only one will take you in the forward direction you need to go in. Only one will lead you to new destinations.

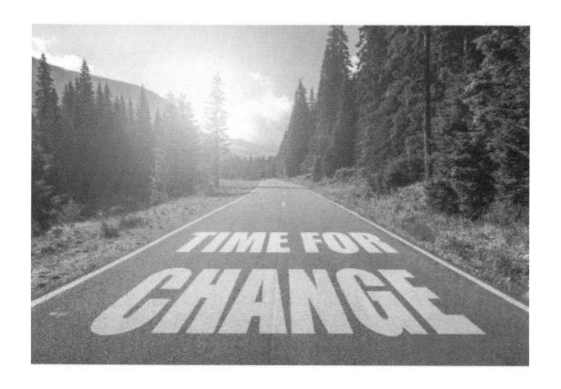

CHANGES

One of the hardest things to do in life is accept change. We get comfortable with our surroundings and environment, even when they no longer fit. Not only is it hard to accept change in our atmosphere, but it is also hard to accept changes within ourselves. Some say that our bodies age every seven years. If our bodies automatically change, we must be comfortable with change all around us.

Unfortunately, a good number of us get comfortable and do not want to change or accept change. Comfort is the enemy of change. How many opportunities have been missed because we were comfortable? Change does not have to be big; it can be a haircut or color, starting a workout, or trying something new to eat. There may be bigger changes you are contemplating, maybe changing careers, buying a home, or starting a business. This week take some moments to think about changes you would like to make in your life, big or small changes. Once you have thought about what changes you would like to make, plan how you will execute the changes. Set a deadline for yourself, so you will be accountable and responsible for your change.

1. What change would you like to make?_____
   _____
   _____

2. What do you need to make the change?_____
   _____
   _____

3. How can you make that change? _____
   _____
   _____

4. What is your deadline? _____
   _____
   _____

∞ ∞ ∞

Scripture verse:
"Therefore, if anyone is in Christ, he is a new creation; old things have passed away; behold, all things have become new."
2 Corinthians 5:17

REMEMBER

C-onstant

H-appenings

A-llow

N-eeded

G-rowth

E-verywhere

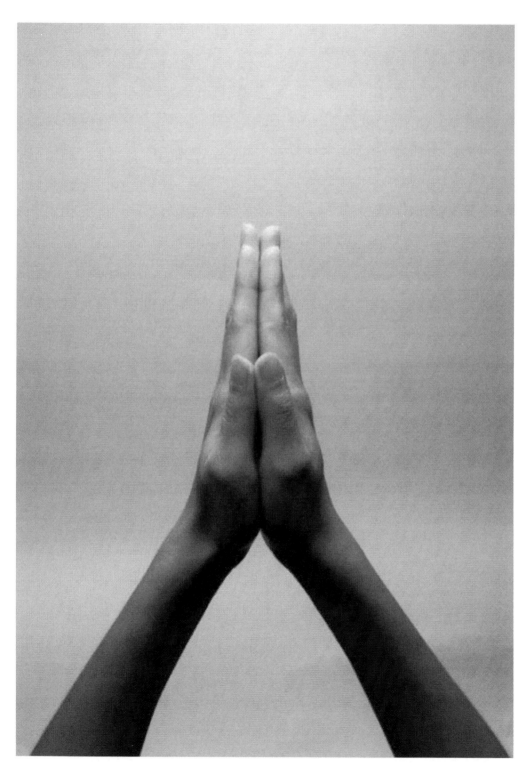

PRAY

There have been tools given to us that will allow us to get answers, release stress, seek wise counsel, cry out for help, lean on someone else besides ourselves, receive guidance, etc. One of those tools is prayer. One thing about prayer that gets overlooked is that prayer is having a dialogue, a two-way conversation, with God. We often treat prayer as a one-sided demand on God. We sometimes use prayer as our last resort instead of our priority. 1 Thessalonians 5:17 tells us to pray without ceasing. So, prayer should never be the last resort, but a tool we always use, not just in times of distress.

I challenge you this week to take at least five minutes to pray. The prayer does not have to be full of fancy words or last a long time. Prayer should come from your heart; it should be real.

1. What would you like to pray about?_____
   _____
   _____

2. Is there anyone you would like to pray for?____
   _____
   _____

3. Are there any issues you need answers for?_____
   _____
   _____

4. What answers did you receive and when?_____
   _____
   _____

∞ ∞ ∞

Scripture verse:
"Therefore I tell you, whatever you ask for in prayer, believe that you have received it, and it will be yours."
Mark 11:24

Prayer Request	Prayer Date	Date Answered

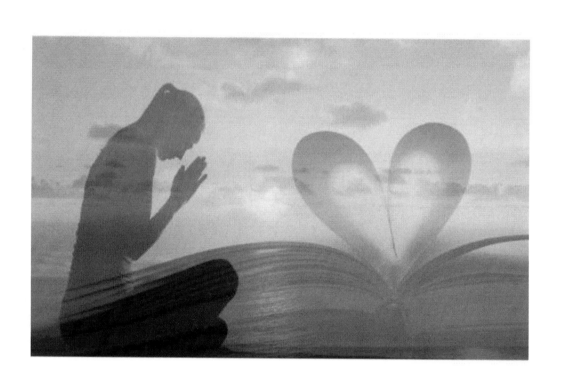

MEDITATE

There are many thoughts about meditation, some positive, some negative. There are many ways to meditate, however, the important factor is to shut down everything on the inside of you and focus on just being. Closing our minds and silencing the noise, is another tool that we can use to find peace, align our thoughts, and repair ourselves. Sometimes sound is important to help us focus. We can use music or sound effects to help slow down the thoughts in our minds. There are scents that can set the atmosphere. There are various incenses, essential oils, candles, sprays, etc., that will heighten awareness. The key is to sit and be still, focus on breathing, and allow yourself to let go.

Meditation is a great way to relieve stress as well. Our minds can get overloaded with information, our bodies can hold on to the pressure of our jobs, family, relationships, etc., and we find ourselves tense and experiencing health issues. Relaxing is key to releasing the tension and anxiety we face daily. There are several books and apps that teach you how to meditate. I challenge you to take 5-15 minutes this week to meditate. Choose a time that is the quietest. Find somewhere where you can be alone. You can sit in a chair, or on the bed, or on the floor; choose somewhere comfortable. Set your atmosphere. Do you want fragrance, do you want sound, do you want light, or do you prefer darkness? Close your eyes. Turn off everything in your mind and focus on your breathing. Take slow, deep breaths, inhale, then exhale. Feel the pressure leave your head, continue to inhale, then exhale. Feel the pressure leave your neck, continue to inhale, then exhale. Feel the pressure leave your shoulders, continue to inhale, then exhale. If thoughts try to enter, do not panic, just focus again on your breathing, breathe in slowly breathe out slowly. Relax in the moment, do not think about what you could/should be doing or what you need to do next. This is not the time to schedule your day. This is about you being still. Continue to breathe until the 5-15 minutes are complete. Try meditating at least three times a week. Do not short yourself on your meditation time, it will be very beneficial to you.

1. How are you feeling? _____
   _____
   _____

2. Is there anything you need to release? _____
   _____
   _____

3. What time is best for you to meditate? _____
   _____
   _____

4. What do you use to meditate? _____
   _____
   _____

∞ ∞ ∞

Scripture verse:
"*He went out to the field one evening to meditate, [a] and as he looked up, he saw camels approaching.*"
Genesis 24:63

DATE OF MEDITATION	LENGTH OF TIME IN MEDITATION	MEDITATION TOOLS (i.e. music, nature sounds, silence, essential oils, incense, etc.)

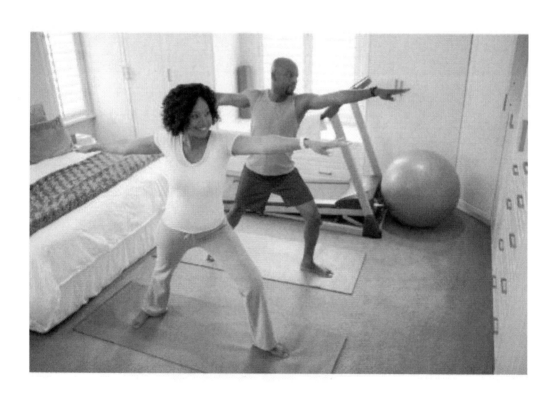

EXERCISE

One-two-three-four, pick those feet up off the floor. Yes, exercise is a huge way for us to care for ourselves. Exercise is personal to you, everyone is different. What might be easy for one person may be very difficult for someone else.

Years ago, I was a trainer at a woman's gym in NJ. I worked out several times a week and was in great shape. Years later, after having my last child, I stopped working out and got caught up in life. I found myself breathing heavily, just walking from my front door to the car parked right out front. I ignored my added weight and inability to walk far for years. I knew I needed to work out, however I was too busy. I was busy working, being a mom, and focusing on other things. Not only was my weight climbing, so was my blood pressure. I still refused to work out and was eventually placed on blood pressure medication. Even being put on medication did not make me want to exercise, I got lazier. I always had an excuse for why I could not start exercising. Even going to the emergency room twice did not push me to work out. It was not until I stepped on the scale one day and saw just how much weight I had picked up, that I started caring. When I tired of clothes no longer fitting and being winded walking up the stairs, that is when I made lifestyle changes.

I did not make myself grand promises, I did not say that I would do 2,500 jumping jacks, run a marathon, or workout for 5 hours a day. I started where I was; I started with something I could do. Instead of parking my car close to the door, I parked a little further away. Instead of walking slowly, I quickened my pace. Doing little things helped me to get comfortable with the thought of working out again. It was also helpful to have accountability partners that were working out too. We would check in daily to see each other's progress.

Some people will need to speak to a doctor and get permission to do a workout program. Some may need to meet with a trainer to get exercise advice. Start out by going to the gym or walking on a track. The choice is yours, however the most important thing you can do is to start and stay the course. Keep going until it becomes a habit, and you find yourself uncomfortable because you did not workout. Your health matters.

1. Will you begin to exercise?_____
   _____
   _____

2. What will be your workout program?_____
   _____
   _____

3. What will be your schedule?_____
   _____
   _____

4. Who will be your accountability partner?_____
   _____
   _____

∞ ∞ ∞

Scripture verse:
"Nevertheless, I will bring health and healing to it; I will heal my people and will let them enjoy abundant peace and security."
Jeremiah 33:6

Date of Exercise	Type of Exercise	Length of Exercise

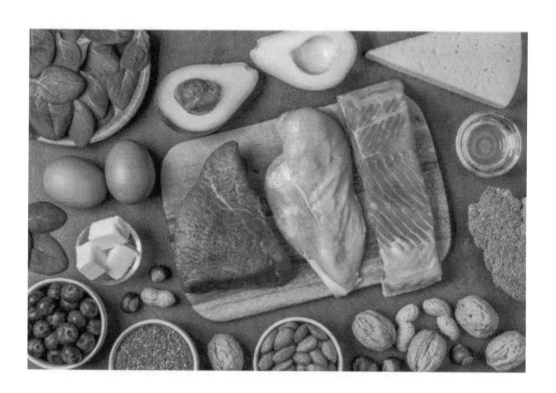

EAT WELL

Eating healthy goes hand in hand with working out. You do not want to do all of that exercising, then fill your body with garbage. You can do an eye roll because I did. I am a chocaholic, I love chocolate. Chips are my second love. Imagine how I felt when my doctor told me both were no-no's for me. Diet is personal to each person. Some people do not eat meat, some eat nothing but seafood. There are many healthy eating programs, many diets, and many fads. Determine what works for you and your body. You may even have to seek advice from a nutritionist or your doctor. Choose what will work for you, not someone else, and be consistent.

1. What are your eating habits now?_____
   _____
   _____

2. What changes do you need to make?_____
   _____
   _____

3. Will you commit to making those changes?_____
   _____
   _____

4. What is your health goal?_____
   _____
   _____

∞ ∞ ∞

Scripture verse:
"*[18] So He said to them, "Are you thus without understanding also? Do you not perceive that whatever enters a man from outside cannot defile him, [19] because it does not enter his heart but his stomach, and is eliminated, [a] thus purifying all foods?"*
Mark 7:18-19

MEAL PLAN

MONDAY	TUESDAY	WEDNESDAY	THURSDAY

FRIDAY	SATURDAY	SUNDAY

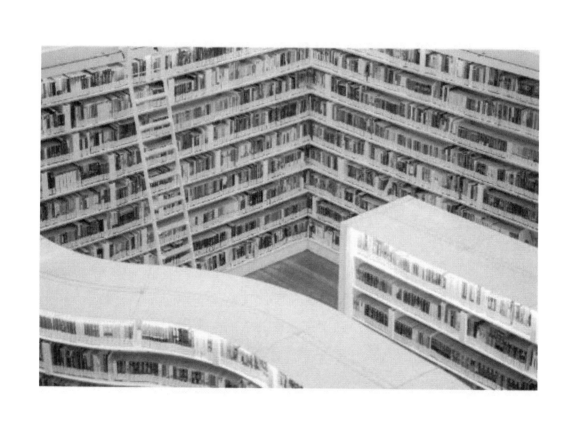

LEARN SOMETHING NEW

You are never too old to learn. We get so caught up in our ages and stages of life, that we close the door on learning something new. Gaining knowledge helps the brain get its exercise. You have wanted to learn a new recipe, why not take a cooking class? You wanted to get your degree, go for it. You wanted to learn how to sew. There are groups that teach sewing, knitting, and crocheting. The only thing that can stop you from doing something new is you. There are online courses, there are even free courses. Now is the perfect time to learn something new.

1. What have you always wanted to learn? _____
   _____
   _____

2. Research where you can study it. _____
   _____
   _____

3. What do you need to enroll? _____
   _____
   _____

4. When will you begin? _____
   _____
   _____

∞ ∞ ∞

Scripture verse:
"Study to shew thyself approved unto God, a workman that needeth not to be ashamed, rightly dividing the word of truth."
2 Timothy 2:15

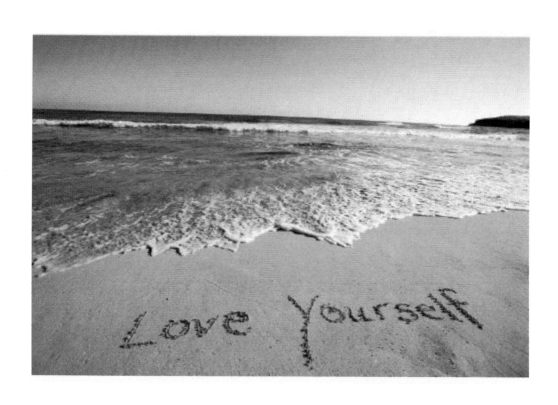

PUT YOURSELF FIRST

You are the best. You are worthy. You are lovely. You are handsome. You are intelligent. You are a Queen. You are a King. You are more than a conqueror. You are the head. Do you take time daily to affirm yourself? Do you love on yourself? There are times we look to others to validate us; however, they are not in a position to validate anyone. We need to know how valuable we are. Sometimes that means we must choose ourselves first. It is hard to pour out to others when you have nothing to pour. When was the last time you put yourself first, put your needs first? You are taking care of family members, children, spouses, loved one, friends, job needs, ministry concerns, bills, household demands, etc. But what about you? What do you need?

1. What do you need? _____
   _____
   _____

2. What decisions do you need to make to better yourself? _____
   _____
   _____

3. How have you affirmed yourself today? _____
   _____
   _____

4. What positive things can you say about yourself? _____
   _____
   _____

∞ ∞ ∞

Scripture verse:
"*I will praise You, for [a]I am fearfully and wonderfully made; Marvelous are Your works, And that my soul knows very well.*"
Psalms 139:14

AFFIRMATIONS

I AM STRESS FREE	MY FINANCES WILL INCREASE
I AM HEALTHY	I WILL NOT GIVE UP
I AM NECESSARY	I AM LOVED
I MATTER	MY HEALTH WILL IMPROVE
I LOVE ME	I FORGIVE OTHERS WHO HAVE HURT ME
I WILL HAVE A WELL-PAID POSITION	I AM BLESSED
I CAN DO GREAT THINGS	MY FAMILY IS WELL
I WILL SUCCEED	TOUGH TIMES WILL END EVENTUALLY
I AM DEBT FREE	MY DREAMS WILL MANIFEST
I WILL FINISH	I WILL LIVE LIFE ABUNDANTLY
I AM COURAGEOUS	THE PERSON GOD HAS FOR ME IS COMING
I WIN	I LOVE THE SKIN THAT I AM IN
I WILL OVERCOME	I WILL PUSH PAST MY FEARS
I AM HEALED	I WILL BE VICTORIOUS
GOD LOVES ME	OBSTACLES WILL MOVE OUT OF MY WAY
I FORGIVE MYSELF	GOD'S GRACE IS ENOUGH
MY RELATIONSHIPS ARE HEALTHY	MY SORROW WILL ONE DAY TURN TO JOY
MY BUSINESS IS GROWING	MY MIND IS CLEAR
CREATIVITY FLOWS FROM ME	I AM BEAUTIFUL/HANDSOME
I WILL CONQUER MY CHALLENGES	I WILL NOT HAVE TO BORROW
I AM ALIVE	I AM WORTHY

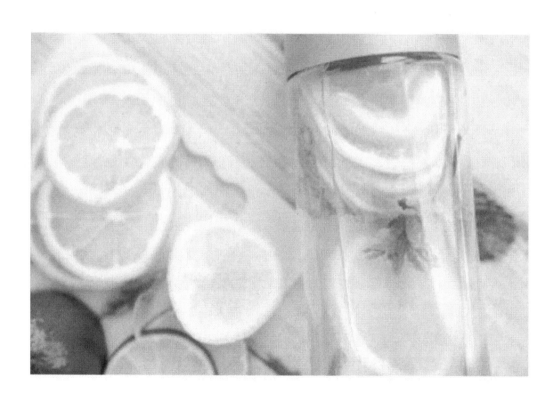

HYDRATE, HYDRATE, HYDRATE

How many of us heard we were made of 60% water in science class? We need to drink water to maintain hydration. Water flushes out toxins and bacteria in our bodies; it is crucial for kidneys and other body functions. Water can aid in weight loss. It also hydrates our skin. I do not know about you, but I want my skin to look younger, not older. There have been various studies done that tell us how much water we should drink. There are those that suggest drinking a gallon of water, some say drink 8 cups of water, while others suggest drinking half your body weight daily. Again, how much water you drink is your choice. As is the kind of water you drink. There are many types of water. There is spring, purified, distilled, and tap, to name a few. And then there are the different brands of water. Do your research to see which kind of water works for you and your health and what taste you like. No, all water does not taste the same. Water should taste good to you so you will enjoy drinking it. Speak to your doctor or a nutritionist to get advice about how much water you should be drinking.

1. Do you drink water? _____
_____
_____

2. How much water do you drink? _____
_____
_____

3. What is your water consumption goal? _____
_____
_____

4. Keep a daily record of how much water you are drinking._____
_____
_____

∞ ∞ ∞

Scripture verse:
"but whoever drinks of the water that I shall give him will never thirst. But the water that I shall give him will become in him a fountain of water springing up into everlasting life."
John 4:14

DATE	WATER (IN OUNCES)

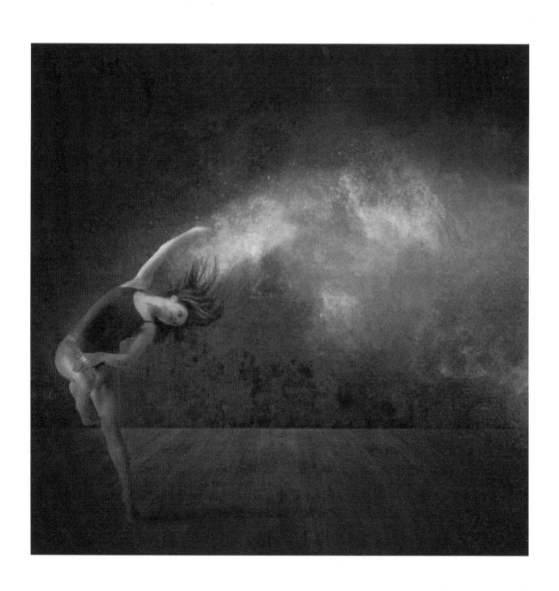

DANCE LIKE NO ONE IS WATCHING

We punch a clock for someone else. We are on highways in horrible traffic. We run to this meeting or that conference. We are soccer moms and dads. We are making dinner and cleaning the house. We make sure our children and pets make it to their various doctor appointments. We are in constant motion, always involved in an activity. There is nothing wrong with being active, however, doing too much will tire us out. Take some minutes a day where you release. Release the hectic activity of your day. One suggestion is to move away from your desk during your lunch. Instead of a working lunch, make it an eating lunch. You will feel much better leaving work for 30-60 minutes and returning to it refreshed. Another suggestion is to take a break during your day and do a fun activity for 15 minutes. It could be coloring, painting, reading, listening to music, dancing around the room, taking a power nap, etc. Taking breaks during your busy day helps to ease a lot of brain fog and lack of focus.

1. What are some quick activities you enjoy?_____
   _____
   _____

2. What activities will you plan for today?_____
   _____
   _____

3. Did you remember to move away from your desk for lunch?_____
   _____
   _____

4. Did you take a break? _____
   _____
   _____

∞ ∞ ∞

Scripture verse:
"You have turned for me my mourning into dancing;
You have put off [a]my sackcloth and clothed me with joy"
Psalm 30:11

5 MINUTE ACTIVITY - Anagrams

Solve.

1. Voices rant on
   _____

2. Dirty room
   _____

3. Salting
   _____

4. Sunlight
   _____

5. Drawback
   _____

6. Moon starer
   _____

7. Amleth
   _____

8. Old West action
   _____

9. Listen
   _____

10.   Nag a ram
   _____

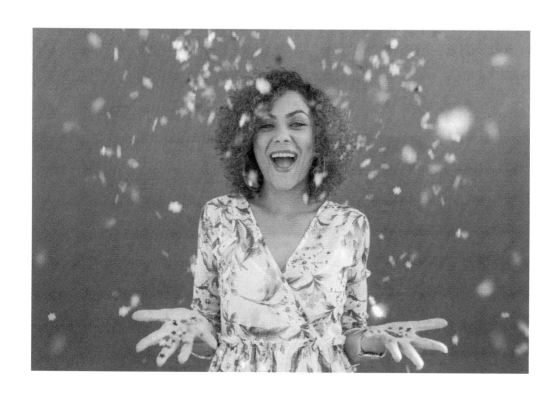

CELEBRATE YOURSELF

Yes, you may have had some failures, yes you may have fallen, however you are still here and still standing. Take some time to focus on your accomplishments. Celebrate you!

1. What have you done that you are happy about?__
   _____
   _____

2. What accomplishment are you most proud of?____
   _____
   _____

3. What failure or struggle have you overcome?___
   _____
   _____

4. What is your greatest strength?_____
   _____
   _____

∞ ∞ ∞

Scripture verse:
"For we are God's handiwork, created in Christ Jesus to do good works, which God prepared in advance for us to do."
Ephesians 2:10

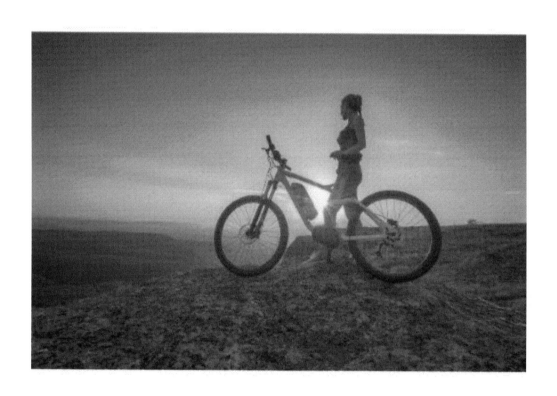

TAKE UP A HOBBY/ACTIVITY

We looked at learning opportunities earlier. Now we will investigate taking up a new hobby or activity. What is something you enjoy doing when you are not working or spending time with your family or friends? You need to have enjoyment in your life. If you do not already have a hobby or an activity that you take part in, choose one that you will spend time on during the next few weeks/months. You may have loved riding a bike, but because of your schedule, hung up your helmet. You may have always wanted to sail a boat, now is the perfect time to do so. Taking time away from the stresses of life is important to maintain your mental and emotional health.

1. What are your current hobbies/activities?_____
   _____
   _____

2. What hobby have you always wanted to do?_____
   _____
   _____

3. Research different hobbies/activities._____
   _____
   _____

4. When will you begin your new hobby/activity?__
   _____
   _____

∞ ∞ ∞

Scripture verse:
"Whatsoever thy hand findeth to do, do it with thy might; for there is no work, nor device, nor knowledge, nor wisdom, in the grave, whither thou goest."
Ecclesiastes 9:10

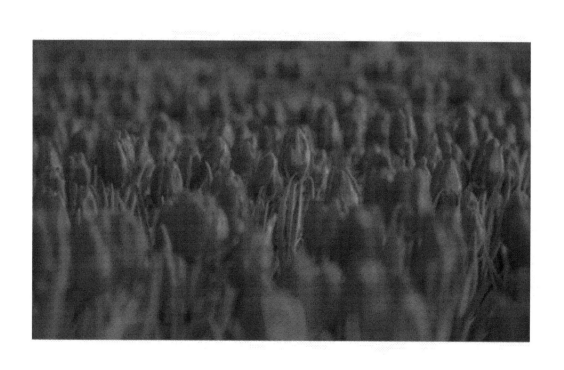

SMELL THE FLOWERS

We get so caught up focusing on the past or fretting about the future, that we forget to live in the moment. You are blessed to be alive right now. Tomorrow will come, but let it come tomorrow. Sure, plan for your future, however, take time to appreciate right where you are. Chew your steak and savor it. Drink your water and let it quench your current thirst. Watch the sun rise and enjoy its brilliance. Treasure each moment you have, now.

1. What is happening in your life currently? _____
   _____
   _____

2. Is there anything affecting you negatively? _____
   _____
   _____

3. How can you turn it into a win? _____
   _____
   _____

4. List something positive that is happening right now. _____
   _____
   _____

∞ ∞ ∞

Scripture verse:
"Therefore do not worry about tomorrow, for tomorrow will worry about itself. Each day has enough trouble of its own."
Matthew 6:34

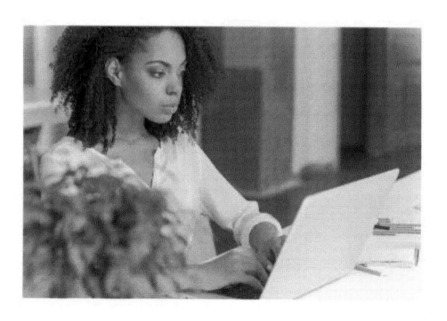

WORK ON PURPOSE

How many of us are working to make someone else's dreams and ambitions come true? How many of us are working on making our own dreams and visions come true? Have you ever asked why you are here? Or do you already know your purpose? There is a time we are to help others build their goals. There is also a time that we must walk into our purpose. If you do not know your purpose, pray, and ask God to reveal it to you. Some say, what hurts you, what makes you cry, reveals your passion and your passion is a part of your purpose. Let me give you an example.

What makes me cry is single mothers, single mothers that cannot afford shelter, utilities, groceries, and essential items. Single mothers that go to get governmental help and the door is closed in their faces hurts me. I have been that single mother many times over. What also hurts me, is the single mother who is at the end of her rope, with no one to help, that does not have a few dollars to spare to drop her children off to a childcare center and take an hour or two to get a facial, a massage, watch a movie, or anything that will help her relax before having to face raising children on her own again. My passion is writing. I want to use my passion and my hurt to walk into my purpose of helping single mothers prosper.

1. What makes you cry?_____
   _____
   _____

2. What is your passion?_____
   _____
   _____

3. What would you do, even if you did not get paid for it, that brings you joy? _____
   _____
   _____

4. How will you walk into your purpose? _____
   _____
   _____

∞ ∞ ∞

Scripture verse:
"*² And the Lord answered me, and said, Write the vision, and make it plain upon tables, that he may run that readeth it. ³ For the vision is yet for an appointed time, but at the end it shall speak, and not lie: though it tarry, wait for it; because it will surely come, it will not tarry.*"
Habakkuk 2:2-3

PURPOSE PLANNER

1 Month Goal	Deadline	Completion Date

List specific things you will do to attain your 1-month goal.

Daily Activity	Weekly Activity

6-Month Goal	Deadline	Completion Date

List specific things you will do to attain your 6-month goal.

Daily Activity	Weekly Activity	Monthly Activity

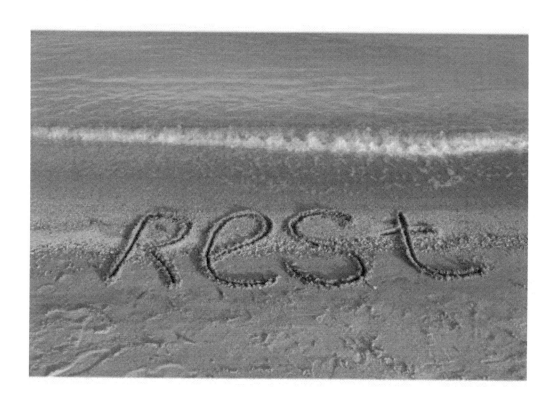

REST

Remember being in preschool and taking naps after eating your lunch and snack? Do you remember how we fought to stay awake because we wanted to talk to our friends? After a while however, we would fall asleep and the teacher would wake us up after what felt like a few minutes and we would feel groggy at first, but soon after, we were full of energy and raring to go. As adults, we need sleep too. Our bodies need sleep to refuel. We cannot miss out on sleep and expect to continue pushing ourselves to the limit. We need both sleep and rest. People often think they are the same, but they are different. Sleep involves your body and conscious mind being inactive, whereas rest is more so being free from pressure, tension, and anxiety. In rest you find peace, calm and tranquility. Rest is necessary to restore you mentally, physically, emotionally, and spiritually.

1. Have you been sleeping?_____
   _____
   _____

2. What keeps you from getting sleep?_____
   _____
   _____

3. Are you rested?_____
   _____
   _____

4. What is causing you not to rest?_____
   _____
   _____

∞ ∞ ∞

Scripture verse:
[28]"*Come to me, all you who are weary and burdened, and I will give you rest.* [29] *Take my yoke upon you and learn from me, for I am gentle and humble in heart, and you will find rest for your souls.* [30] *For my yoke is easy and my burden is light."*
Matthew 11:28-30

SLEEP JOURNAL - MORNING

	Sun	Mon	Tues	Wed	Thurs	Fri	Sat
Bedtime (Last Night)							
Wake-Up Time (This Morning)							
Amount of Time to Fall Asleep							
# of Times You Woke During the Night							
# of Total Hours You Slept							
Did anything interrupt your sleep?							
How would you rate your sleep (from 1-5_							
How do you feel this morning?							
Comments							

SLEEP JOURNAL - NIGHT

	Sun	Mon	Tues	Wed	Thurs	Fri	Sat
How many caffeinated drinks did you have today?							
Have you taken any medications today?							
Did you work out today?							
Did you take a nap today?							
How many alcoholic drinks did you have today?							
Today did you feel: Stressed Cranky Drained Sick Irritable							
Did you have a headache?							
Were you able to focus?							
Did you eat late?							
Did you have a							

good day?							
Comments							

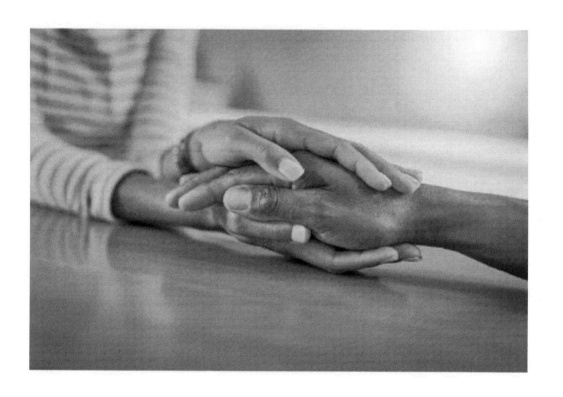

HELP SOMEONE ELSE

The feeling of helping someone else is unmatched. In Acts 20:35, the Bible tells us "that it is more blessed to give than receive." The Bible also tells us in 2 Corinthians 9:7 that "God loves a cheerful giver." What should we give to others? We should give our time, our talents, and our treasures.

Giving of our time may be a sacrifice especially when we have full plates already, however, calling to check on someone, taking someone to the store, serving meals to the homeless, or caring for a loved one are times well spent and self-rewarding.

Giving of our talents can sometimes be daunting, we want to be compensated for what we are skilled, blessed, and talented to do. However, there are times we will do a great service for someone by offering our talents for free. Are you great at math? You could offer tutoring to a neighborhood child who is struggling in that area. Are you gifted to sing? You could offer to sing at the nursing home once a month, to uplift the residents. Are you a skilled seamstress or tailor? You can provide a prom gown or tuxedo for youth who cannot afford clothing for their prom. We are all gifted to do something, from time to time we can extend our gifting for free.

Our treasure is our money. Most of us are okay with giving our time and talents to others, but with our hard-earned money, we push back. After all, don't we have bills to pay, families to support, and dreams to achieve? We have stretched the dollar to within an inch of it breaking. How can we afford to give our money to someone or something else? We get indignant sometimes, don't we? "Why can't they get a job?" "I worked hard for my money; they should work just as hard." "They need to stop being lazy." "I just gave to the building fund, here they are begging for something else." "How do I know that they are going to do the right thing with my money?" The truth is we do not know what people will do with the money we give. They may misuse it, they may use it in a different area than what they told us, or they may use it in the manner they said they would. Our job is not to delegate how money we give is used. Our job is to give as we are led to give and then wash our hands of it. If we have it, if God placed it in our spirits to give, then give it without a second thought. Proverbs 19:17 tells us "Whoever is generous to the poor lends to the Lord, and He will repay him for his deed." My dad gave me sage advice when I was a young girl. He told me to never lend money, instead give it. He said that if I could not afford to lose it, then to not give it. He lived with that principle his entire life and he never stressed about who owed him money, because he gave money, never lent it.

You may not think your treasure will be a blessing because you do not have a lot to give, however every bit helps. When my oldest daughter was just six or seven years old, we were in dire straits. We had no food, and my paycheck was not coming for a week. I did not know what I was going to do because I only had $3 left to spend. I went to church, and the message was uplifting, it gave me hope. I put the last $3 I had in the offering plate, not knowing how I would survive the week, needing gas and food. After service I ran into a very close friend of mine, she is my adopted aunt. She checked in with us, asked if we were okay and if we were hungry. My pride would not let me tell her I had no food in the house, and that I had not eaten that day. She headed back to the church and as my daughter got in the car, she turned back and said that God had just put me in her spirit, and she handed me something folded up. When I opened it, it was money, more money than I needed to fill my tank up and buy food for a week. Tears streamed down my face and I felt a relief I had not felt in months. She apologized and said she wished she could have done more. What she thought was little, was much to me. You sowing when God puts it into your spirit can save someone's life. Giving your time, talent and treasure is not only a blessing to the person/people you are blessing, but it blesses you too.

1. When was the last time you helped someone?_____
   _____
   _____

2. Has anyone ever blessed you? How did it make you feel?_____
_____
_____

3. Who is in your spirit to help?_____
_____
_____

4. How did helping them make you feel?_____
_____
_____

∞ ∞ ∞

Scripture verse:
"not looking to your own interests but each of you to the interests of the others."
Philippians 2:4

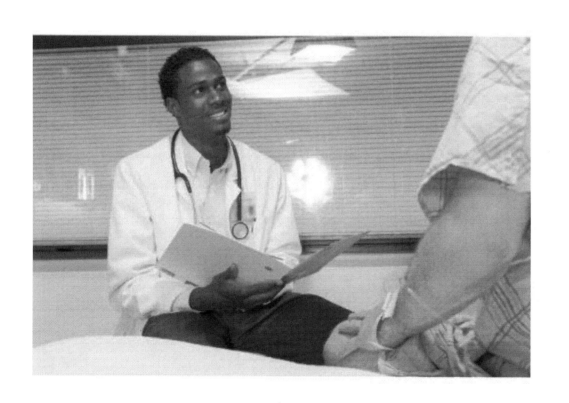

GET A CHECK UP

We have spoken a lot about checking with our nutritionists and doctors to get advice. It is very hard to check in with them about diet, exercise, and water intake if we do not go for regularly scheduled visits. We have begun a dangerous practice of self-diagnosing and self-prescribing. When we feel under the weather, we will go to the internet to see what ailment lines up with our symptoms. I understand that a lot of us cannot go to the doctor, dentist, or optometrist because we neither have insurance nor money to go. If you can go, it is important to that you do. Early detection of anything gives a better opportunity for it to be treated and healed.

1. How are you feeling?_____
   _____
   _____

2. When was the last time you were seen by a doctor, dentist, and optometrist?_____
   _____
   _____

3. Are you following their recommendations?_____
   _____
   _____

4. When is your next appointment?_____
   _____
   _____

∞ ∞ ∞

Scripture verse:
"So we do not lose heart. Though our outer self[a] is wasting away, our inner self is being renewed day by day."
2 Corinthians 4:16

NO NEGATIVITY ALLOWED HERE

RELEASE NEGATIVITY AND NEGATIVE PEOPLE

One of the biggest destroyers of our peace is negativity. There is nothing like walking into your home after a long day of work and walking on eggshells, fearful that your significant other, children, family members or roommate has had a bad day and will meet you with a negative attitude. There is no worse feeling than having something great happen to you, but when you share it, it is ignored, downplayed, or ripped apart. Unfortunately, there are many of us who have negative people around us. They come in the form of parents, siblings, children, friends, employers, co-workers, spiritual leaders, neighbors, etc. Anyone can be a negative influence in your life.

It is hard to counterattack negativity, however it is possible. Its purpose is to steal your joy, rob your ambition, kill your passion, and destroy your dreams. However, realizing your power, authority, and capability, crushes its power over you. Speaking to negativity with positivity eliminates it. Removing negative people from your circle is important. Releasing some people is easier than others. It may not be possible to detach from some family members, friends, employers, or co-workers, completely, however you can limit your time around them. You can also shut down negative conversations. There is nothing wrong with securing your peace.

When we are the source of negativity, we must feed ourselves positivity. Instead of saying what you cannot do, say what you can do. Instead of putting yourself down, uplift yourself. You must focus more on the positive than the negative. I challenge you this week, start with one hour per day, to speak nothing but positivity to yourself and others.

1. What negative people do you need to release? __
   _____
   _____

2. What negative words do you need to release about yourself? _____
   _____
   _____

3. Were you able to be positive for at least one hour every day this week? _____
   _____
   _____

4. How can you be more positive? _____
   _____
   _____

∞ ∞ ∞

Scripture verse:
"Warn a divisive person once, and then warn them a second time. After that, have nothing to do with them."
Titus 3:10

How to Counteract Negative Emotions

- Hatred --------------------------------Love
  "Do everything in love." 1 Corinthians 16:14
- Misery ---------------------------------Joy
  "Count it all joy, my brothers, when you meet trials of various kinds." James 1:2
- Conflict -------------------------------Peace
  "Peace I leave with you; My peace I give you. Not as the world gives do I give it to you. Let not your hearts be troubled, neither let them be afraid." John 14:27
- Impatience -----------------------------Patience
  "You almost must be patient. Keep your hopes high, for the day of the Lord is coming near." James 5:8
- Cruelty/Meanness -----------------------Kindness
  "A man who is kind benefits himself, but a cruel man hurts himself." Proverbs 11:17
- Wickedness/Evil ------------------------Goodness
  "Do not be overcome by evil, but overcome evil with good." Romans 12:21
- Faithlessness/Disloyalty ---------------Faithfulness
  "And if you faithfully obey the voice of the Lord your God, being careful to do all His commandments that I command you today, the Lord your God will set you high above all the nations of the earth. And all these blessings shall come upon you and overtake you, if you obey the voice of the Lord your God. Deuteronomy 28:1-2
- Harshness/Hard Heartedness -------------Gentleness
  "Refuse to get involved in inane discussions; they always end up in fights. God's servant must not be argumentative, but a gentle listener and a teacher who keeps cool, working firmly but patiently with those who refuse to obey." - 2 Timothy 2:23-25
- Indulgence -----------------------------Self-Control
  "People who cannot control themselves are like cities without walls to protect them." - Proverbs 25:28
- [22] But the fruit of the Spirit is love, joy, peace, patience, kindness, goodness, faithfulness, [23] gentleness, self-control; against such things there is no law.

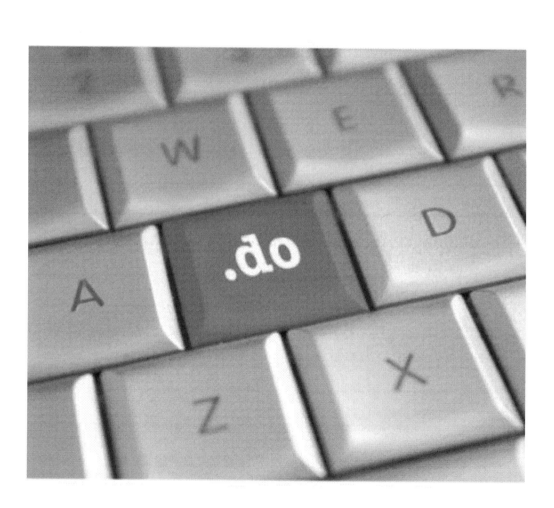

DO SOMETHING YOU'VE ALWAYS WANTED

We put off doing things until we retire or have saved more than enough money to do it. The problem is that when we keep putting things off, there is less likelihood that it will happen.

"I will go when flights are cheaper."

"I will do it after this project."

"I will do it when I get my life together."

What happens? After we complete one project, another comes along. When the flights get cheaper, we have to use the money for a repair to the house. When do we ever completely get our lives together? Something always comes up, and something always happens. We must live for today. That does not mean to shuck responsibility and neglect work or your other duties.

At the beginning of the year, my children and I make a list, of three-five things we will focus on for the entire year. We are very specific, whether it is getting an "A" on a test or traveling to a certain place, we keep those as our focuses all year and we are accountable to each other. If our focus item requires money, then we put money aside until we have the amount we need and that money is only for that item, no matter what happens. My great-aunt taught me a great principle. It is the pay yourself principle. After tithing, she told me to take another 10% out of my income and put it aside in an envelope or jar marked "Self". The "Self" money is only for you to do something you want. This is not to be confused with "rainy day" money. Rainy day money goes for anything that you might need money for. Your "Self" money is strictly for you to do something for yourself.

We must get over thinking we do not deserve what we want. You have worked hard all your life, yes you deserve a bag from a name brand designer, if you can afford it. Yes, you deserve a trip to Brazil, Africa, Jamaica, or wherever you want to go, if you can afford it. Do not live beyond your means, however, live. If you want to go on a trip, for example, you can use the pay yourself principle, or start a trip fund and save 2-5% of your check to go towards it. This fund will not be for car repairs, or any other emergency that comes up. Put this fund out of your thoughts. It is only to be added to and used for its purpose.

1. What have you been putting off that you want to do?_____
_____
_____

2. How will you make time to do it?_____
_____
_____

3. Do you have the money to do it?_____
_____
_____

4. Put together a plan to do it within the next 12 months._____
_____
_____

∞ ∞ ∞

Scripture verse:
"*May he give you the desire of your heart and make all your plans succeed.*"
Psalm 20:4

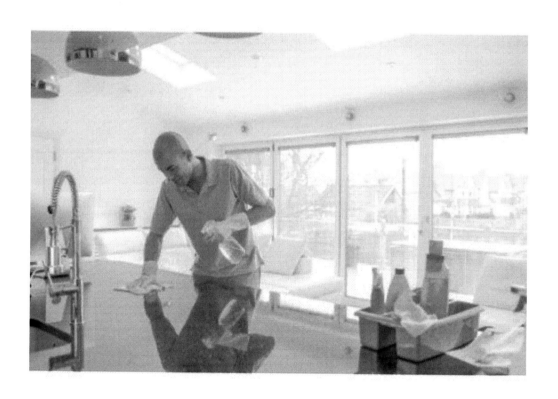

CLEAN OUT YOUR CLOSET

Spring brings on the feelings of warmer days, green trees, and cleaning. It is usually the time of year people clean their homes from top to bottom. In our lives we go through many emotions, many feelings, many realities, disappointments, and hurts. We walk around carrying baggage instead of letting it go. We go into new relationships with old pain. We begin new friendships with old betrayal. We join new churches with old hurt. We start new jobs with old disappointments. Often, we do not even realize all the negativity and bitterness spewing out of us because of unresolved issues. A few pages ago we discussed forgiveness, and the great relief that true forgiveness brings. Now we will discuss how dusting out the cobwebs of unresolved issues will help us walk into true release.

You have forgiven the person, you have moved on, but why does your significant other not answering their phone when you call the first time set you off. Why do you become so impatient when your new friend tells you to hold on? Why do you rush out of the church as soon as the doors open? Why do you refuse to meet people, talk to people or join any of the ministries of the church? Why do you roll your eyes and get irritated every time your new supervisor asks to meet with you? A lot of us have forgiven people and forgiven situations but held on to a remnant of what they did to us. We remember vividly that John used to ignore our calls, and we discovered he was cheating. We think back to the times Jamie put us on hold to talk about us to someone on her other line. We feel the resurfaced pain of how Sister Gladys and Mother Jenkins talked down to us when we served in the missions' ministry at our old church. We recall how Mr. Barber called us into his office to harp on a mistake we made or to tell us we were unqualified for our job. John, Jamie, Sister Gladys, Mother Jenkins, and Mr. Barber have all been forgiven, however we still feel the leftover effects of pain, betrayal, hurt and disappointment.

We must deal with the residue of these leftover emotions. It is not fair that you enter a new relationship, a new friendship, or a new opportunity with bitterness and resentment from something or someone from your past. They deserve a clean slate and a fresh start. This is a good time for you to do spring cleaning on yourself. Examine yourself for any hurt, pain, feelings of betrayal, disappointment, resentment, anger, distrust, or any other negative emotion. Now that you know what negative emotions you are dealing with, pray and ask God to release you from them. You may need to speak to the person/people from your past so that you can have closure. You may have to confront some things you were unwilling to face before. There might be unresolved emotions because you refused to deal with the situation openly, honestly, and completely. When something is painful, we tend to sweep it under the rug. If we keep sweeping things under the rug, they eventually pile up and become too large to cover up. When you have confronted the issues of your past, it is time to make amends with those that are connected to you in the present. Discuss the negative things you were saying or doing to the person/people presently in your life. It helps to be open and honest with your feelings.

"Aaron, I apologize for snapping at you the other day when you did not answer my call. I will try not to act that way again. I realize you are not my ex."

Then you can discuss how you are letting go of some past pain.

"Marie, I apologize for hanging up on you the other day and then ignoring your calls and texts. Putting me on hold for long periods of time reminded me of a bad experience I had with a former friend."

Attempt to not punish the new people in your life for acts that your former connections did. Being in a relationship, no matter if it is personal or professional, requires you to have honest communication and to be open.

"Hello Anne, it's great to meet you. I am interested in the missions' ministry here; I would like to get better acquainted with the policies of the church and the ministry."

"Good morning Ms. James, I see you have the presentation I created. Is it okay or are there some changes you can suggest?"

By confronting your negative emotions and taking the lead on being open, you bypass the power the unresolved issues had over you. This will not guarantee that Aaron is not cheating, or Marie is not talking behind your back, or that you will not have the same issues at your new church or job, however each new person and opportunity need to be given the chance to start off fresh without riding the coattails of the negative actions in your past.

1. What are you holding on to?_____
   _____
   _____

2. Have you or are you treating someone unfairly?
   _____
   _____
   _____

3. What do you need to change? _____
   _____
   _____

4. How can you make those changes? _____
   _____
   _____

∞ ∞ ∞

Scripture verse:
"*³¹ Get rid of all bitterness, rage and anger, brawling and slander, along with every form of malice. ³² Be kind and compassionate to one another, forgiving each other, just as in Christ God forgave you.*"
Ephesians 4:31-32

SPRING CLEANING CHECKLIST

- ☐ Empty out all your negative emotions and feelings about the situation/person (This may include praying, speaking to a trusted confidant, writing in your journal, speaking to the source, writing a letter, etc.)
- ☐ Air out your emotions. Get out all your tears, sadness, anger, frustration, etc.
- ☐ Dust off those hidden emotions. It is time to shine a light on your true feelings, the ones you hide from everyone else (i.e. the smiles that hide the tears, the fancy clothes, and bags, that hide your tattered and torn heart)
- ☐ Rip out the situation from the root, do not let anything remain
- ☐ Remove any and everything that reminds you of the situation (It is time to declutter)
- ☐ Throw out letters, pictures, delete emails, text messages and voicemails regarding the situation/person
- ☐ After you have thrown out/gotten rid of everything it is time to organize what you have left (What feelings are left? What emotions do you have? Have you physically deleted/thrown out everything that leaves you feeling bitter, resentful, etc.? Have you let go?)
- ☐ It is cleaning time! Ask God to renew your mind and spirit. Pamper yourself today (take a nice, long bath, go to the spa, get your favorite treat, etc.) you have made a major accomplishment
- ☐ Flip your emotions, you have gotten rid of the negativity, now focus on the positive. What do you have going on in your life that is positive?
- ☐ Wipe off your dreams, hopes and goals. It is time to walk into your calling/purpose/assignment
- ☐ Reseal your relationship with yourself, let no one and nothing throw you off track from moving forward into destiny
- ☐ Sprinkle words of affirmation over yourself daily
- ☐ Clean off your testimony to use to help someone else overcome

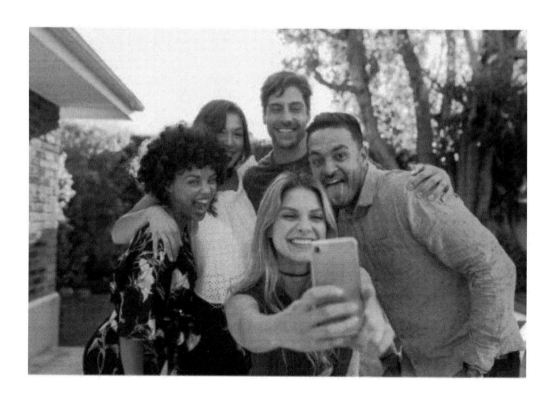

JOIN UP WITH FRIENDS

We have life going on. We are active at work or in business, we have families to maintain, children to raise, we have chores, we may be in school, etc. We realize that our plates are full, however we all need time to unwind and be around other people we like. Friends provide an outlet for conversation, laughter, and fun. As busy as you are still schedule time with friends. We all need to push away from our lives for a moment and be around like-minded people, that have our best interest at heart. You may have friends you just go to concerts with, friends you go out to eat with, friends you play games with, or friends you seek advice and wise counsel from. There are some friends you can do all those things with. Dedicate at least one night a month to hang out with your friends. You will feel better for it.

1. Do you have a close friend?_____
   _____
   _____

2. When was the last time you spoke to your friend?
   _____
   _____
   _____

3. Have you scheduled a time to meet up?_____
   _____
   _____

∞ ∞ ∞

Scripture verse:
"not giving up meeting together, as some are in the habit of doing, but encouraging one another—and all the more as you see the Day approaching."
Hebrews 10:25

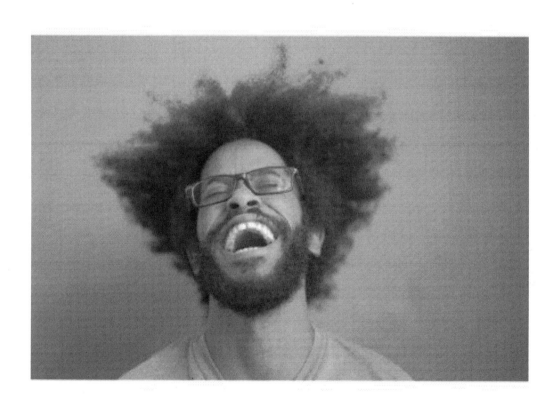

LAUGH

What is your favorite comedy? What is one thing that always makes you laugh? Laughter is healing, and it has also been said that laughter is an excellent form of stress relief. Take time out of your day to laugh. Think of a joke, listen to a comedy station, or watch your favorite comedian. Laugh, laugh, laugh!

1. List a funny memory you have. _____
   _____
   _____

2. What is the last thing that caused you to have a deep belly laugh? _____
   _____
   _____

3. When was the last time you smiled? When was the last time you laughed? _____
   _____
   _____

4. What movie, tv show or book makes you laugh?
   _____
   _____
   _____

∞ ∞ ∞

Scripture verse:
"Our mouths were filled with laughter, our tongues with songs of joy. Then it was said among the nations, "The Lord has done great things for them."
Psalm 126:2

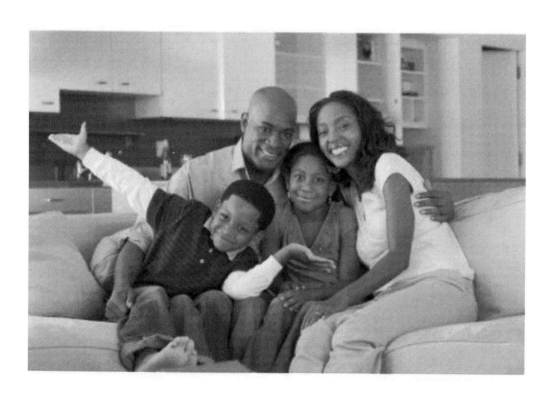

SPEND TIME WITH FAMILY

Family can uplift us, they can disappoint us, they can heal us, or they can cause pain. Most of us could not choose our families, but God gave them to us. If there is any family trauma, please try to heal and forgive it. Life is short and you do not want to regret having a rift in your family. All families are not the same, so do not compare yours to another as a standard. You never want unforgiveness to cause you to miss the opportunity to spend time with those you love.

1. Do you have family trauma?_____
   _____
   _____

2. Are you able to forgive it?_____
   _____
   _____

3. What do you love about your family?_____
   _____
   _____

4. When is the next time you will spend time with your family?_____
   _____
   _____

∞ ∞ ∞

Scripture verse:
"Bear with one another and, if one has a complaint against another, forgive each other; as the Lord has forgiven you, so you also must forgive."
Colossians 3:13

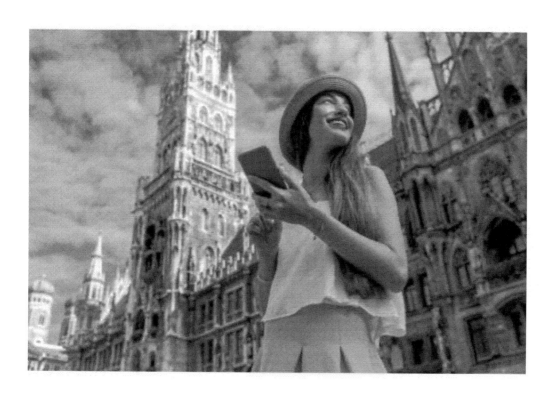

TRAVEL

Getting away from it all can be very therapeutic. Leaving behind the strains and pressures of your home life and taking time to go visit somewhere different can be a great stress reliever. I have found that cleaning up before leaving for vacation helps ease distress when you return. If you have family members that are not traveling with you, give them the fun task of making sure everything is in order.

While you are away be a tourist and enjoy the local sites and activities. I had a friend who went away to a tropical paradise and stayed in the hotel room the entire time; they saw nothing of the country and complained that they had a rotten time. I would not suggest over packing your vacation with activities either. Another friend went away and had activities scheduled from the time they woke until they closed their eyes. When they got back home, they needed a vacation from the vacation. You want to balance your time away.

Vacations do not have to be major trips away. You can stay at a local hotel and enjoy the amenities. For many years, my children and I have gone to a local resort for a weekend getaway and have enjoyed room service, the pools, and the local activities, as if we did not live 20 minutes away. You can even turn your own home into a vacation stay. I do not suggest taking work on vacation or answering too many calls and texts. The point is to get away from your current life happenings, to relax your body and your mind, and to have fun.

1. Where will your next adventure be?_____
_____
_____

2. What is your dream vacation? _____
   _____
   _____

3. Plan your next vacation to take place within a year of today, even if it is only to a local hotel. _____
   _____
   _____

∞ ∞ ∞

Scripture verse:
"By day the Lord went ahead of them in a pillar of cloud to guide them on their way and by night in a pillar of fire to give them light, so that they could travel by day or night."
Exodus 13:21

TRAVEL ITINERARY

Start Date:

End Date:

Destination:

FLIGHT DETAILS				
Flight Details	Date	Airline(s)	Arrival Time	Terminal

HOTEL DETAILS				
Check In	Hotel	Address	Inclusion	Check Out

DAY 1	
TIME	ACTIVITY

DAY 2	
TIME	ACTIVITY

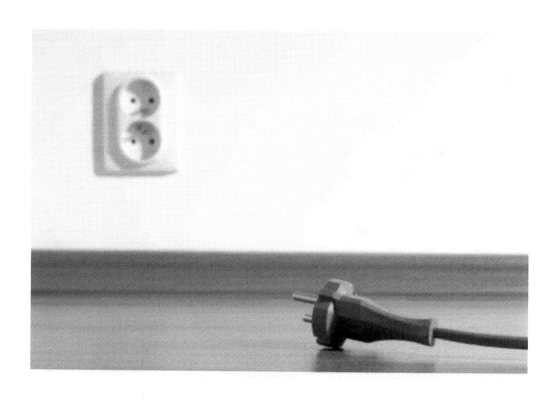

UNPLUG

Turn everything off. Shut down your computer. Turn off your cell phone, watch, tablet, game system, television, radio, e-book device, and social media. You are now unplugged from the world. Take at least one hour to just be. Do not worry about that paper that is due, the bills you were about to pay, the dinner you were about to make, or the work you brought home from the office. Shut off all activities for one hour and check on yourself. Take this time to pray, meditate, journal, nap, or be still. It is in this quiet time that you may hear answers to questions you have had or think of something new you want to do. Practice unplugging at least once a week.

1. How are you feeling? _____
   _____
   _____

2. Is there anything affecting you? _____
   _____
   _____

3. Have you discovered a solution to a situation?
   _____
   _____
   _____

4. Have you come up with a creative idea? _____
   _____
   _____

∞ ∞ ∞

Scripture verse:
"Do not conform to the pattern of this world, but be transformed by the renewing of your mind."
Romans 12:2

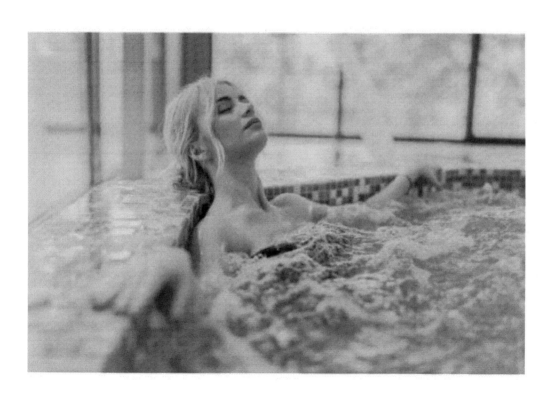

PAMPER YOURSELF

There is nothing like being pampered. We all deserve to pamper ourselves. Whether you like massages, spa treatments, facials, getting your hair done, manicures, pedicures, or other types of pampering, try to have a pampering day a few times a month. This is another way to release tension and let go of stress and anxiety. There are apps online and in your smartphone's store area that offer discounts on everything from exotic lunches to hot stone massages and acupuncture.

Pampering does not have to be expensive. Pampering could be spending "me" time with yourself doing what you want to do, taking a nice warm bath, bingeing your favorite tv show, taking a nap, having your favorite drink or treat, listening to your favorite music, coloring, painting, writing, or reading a book. If you are enjoying yourself, that is considered pampering.

1. What soothes you?_____
   _____
   _____

2. What do you like doing?_____
   _____
   _____

3. What ways will you pamper yourself this month?
   _____
   _____
   _____

4. What have you never tried that you would like to try?_____
   _____
   _____

∞ ∞ ∞

Scripture verse:
"With promises like this to pull us on, dear friends, let's make a clean break with everything that defiles or distracts us, both within and without."
2 Corinthians 7:1

Today I am grateful for

HAVE AN ATTITUDE OF GRATITUDE

One of the best ways to love on yourself is to remember the things you have been through and how you overcame them. My cousin challenged us to write something we were thankful for everyday for a year, and at the end of the year look through the book at everything we had written and remember how we had been blessed. Another challenge is to write your request/prayer on a piece of paper, the date you are writing the request, and hang it on the wall. When the request/prayer is answered, write the date the request is answered and how it was answered, then put the paper in a jar and keep it. When you are having a bad day, going through a struggle, or feeling low, open the jar and pull out one sheet and be reminded of how God answered you.

Count your blessings and know how blessed you truly are.

1. What are you grateful for?_____
   _____
   _____
   _____
   _____
   _____
   _____
   _____
   _____
   _____

∞ ∞ ∞

Scripture verse:
"This is the day which the Lord has made;
Let's rejoice and be glad in it."
Psalm 118:24

SELF CHECK

1. How do you feel right now?
   _____
   _____
   _____

2. What successes did you have today?
   _____
   _____
   _____

3. What failures did you have today?
   _____
   _____
   _____

4. How can you turn your failures into positive outcomes? _____
   _____
   _____
   _____

5. What inspires you?
   _____
   _____
   _____

6. What one thing do you dream of doing/having?
   _____
   _____
   _____

7. How can you make that dream a reality?
_____
_____
_____

8. What do you need to forgive yourself for?
_____
_____
_____

9. Are you hurting? _____
_____
_____

10. How can that hurt be healed?
_____
_____
_____

11. What are you doing that is wasteful?
_____
_____
_____

12. What can you do to further your goals?
_____
_____
_____

13. What did you do that made you smile today?
_____
_____
_____

14. Did you exercise this week?
   _____
   _____
   _____

15. Did you eat something healthy today?
   _____
   _____
   _____

16. Did you work on something that will better your future?_____
   _____
   _____

17. Did you speak more positivity than negativity today?_____
   _____
   _____

18. Who did you help today?_____
   _____
   _____

19. Did you pray today?_____
   _____
   _____

20. Did you meditate this week?
   _____
   _____
   _____

21. What hobby have you started/planned to start?
   _____
   _____
   _____

22. What have you said to affirm yourself today?
   _____
   _____
   _____

23. Did you contact a family member or friend to check on them? _____
   _____
   _____

24. What learning project have you begun or plan to begin? _____
   _____
   _____

25. What one thing are you grateful for you?
   _____
   _____
   _____

26. In this present moment what do you see, hear, smell, taste and feel? _____
   _____
   _____

27. Have you gone to the doctor / dentist / optometrist in the last year?
_____
_____
_____

28. Have you cleaned out your closet?
_____
_____
_____

29. What have you checked off your always wanted to do list?_____
_____
_____

30. What did you do to pamper yourself?
_____
_____
_____

31. Have you removed negativity from your life?
_____
_____
_____

ABOUT THE AUTHOR

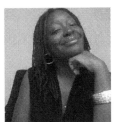

Andrea Joyce, is a native of New Jersey, currently living in Atlanta, Georgia.
She is the proud mother of one son and two daughters.
Besides writing books, Andrea enjoys writing, directing, and producing
for stage and screen.
Visit her online at www.authorandreajoyce.weebly.com or email her at
authorandreajoyce@gmail.com.